CANCER FIGHTING FEASTS

HOW TO FIGHT CANCER WITH EASY AND NOURISHING RECIPES

RYAN STONE

TABLE OF CONTENT

Introduction

There are strands of laughter, love, and joy sewn into the fabric of life. However, certain threads are also characterised by difficulty, unexpectedness, and challenge. I entered the world of cancer-fighting feasts at a critical juncture that will always be marked in my memory as a time of both suffering and resolve.

In summer 2017, everything in my world seemed to be out of balance. My grandmother, a force to be reckoned with in our family, was given the news we all dread: cancer. She was a colourful, independent woman. Her laughter, which used to fill our house, was now mingled with the quiet murmurs of hospital hallways.

The one thing that remained constant while we made our way through the maze of visits, treatments, and uncertainty was our kitchen. Motivated by my grandmother's unwavering will, I set out to prepare meals that would nourish her body while it fought this powerful foe, in addition to satisfying her appetite.

During those moments in the kitchen, a new story emerged—one of resiliency, optimism, and the transforming potential of healthful food. Cancer Fighting Feasts is more than simply a cookbook—it's a record of our family's culinary adventure and evidence of our conviction that every lovingly prepared meal is a tiny triumph over the evils of disease.

Imagine, as you turn the pages of these pages, a kitchen full of the sound of pots and pans clattering, spices dancing all around, and laughter that laughs at the ridiculousness of our circumstances. I sincerely hope that this book serves as a beacon of hope for you as it is a testimony to the amazing trip that my family took.

Come along on this culinary journey with me, where each dish is a chapter of resiliency and each recipe is a page turned in the story of recovery. Cancer Fighting Feasts is about transforming common materials into remarkable tales of resilience, fortitude, and the enduring strength of the human spirit. Welcome to a kitchen where love is the unshakable beauty of life and every dish is an expression of that beauty.

Kitchen Essentials for Cancer-Fighting Recipes

The kitchen is the centre of every home and a haven of healing and sustenance. It is impossible to overestimate the significance of having a well-equipped kitchen as we navigate the terrain of creating cancer-fighting meals. This chapter serves as your manual, giving you a thorough rundown of the kitchen necessities to enable you to prepare healthful meals that are infused with the fortitude required to combat illness.

1. Vibrant and Fresh Produce:

Fresh fruits and vegetables with their brilliant colours are the foundation of dishes that fight cancer. These vibrant jewels are the mainstay of a diet that fortifies the body against the effects of cancer since they are packed with antioxidants, vitamins, and minerals. A produce section full of fresh food, from leafy greens to berries loaded with phytochemicals, is your first port of call.

2. Whole Legumes and Grains:

Whole grains and legumes are generally considered healthful foods that form the basis of a well-balanced plate. Packed with dietary fibre, these nutrients support healthy digestion and help keep blood sugar levels steady. These pantry mainstays, which range from quinoa and brown rice to lentils and chickpeas, give your cancer-fighting recipe arsenal more substance and nutritional depth.

3. Trim Proteins:

Since proteins are the building blocks of life, choosing lean sources is essential when creating recipes to combat cancer.

Include lean meats, fish, tofu, and chicken without the skin to guarantee a diet high in protein and low in unneeded saturated fats. These protein sources are essential for helping the body heal damaged tissue and bolstering the immune system.

4. Healthy Fats:
Acknowledge the power of fats that come from nuts, seeds, avocados, and olive oil. These fats support heart health generally in addition to giving your food a delicious richness. Salmon and other fatty fish are rich sources of omega-3 fatty acids, which have anti-inflammatory qualities and are especially helpful when it comes to nutrition that fights cancer.

5. Spices and Herbs:
Using a variety of herbs and spices will help your cancer-fighting meals taste better. Many herbs and spices have

anti-inflammatory and antioxidant qualities in addition to their gastronomic appeal. These taste enhancers are also health companions in your kitchen, from fresh herbs like basil and rosemary to turmeric with its curcumin content.

6. High-Nutrient Drinks:

Don't undervalue the importance of drinks in your battle against cancer. Herbal infusions and green tea, which is renowned for its high antioxidant content, can make delicious complements to your daily hydration regimen. Maintaining adequate hydration is essential, and adding nutrition to your drinks is an easy yet effective way to do this.

7. Tools for Preparing Meals:

A kitchen that is well-stocked is incomplete without the appropriate tools.

Invest in high-quality cookware, chopping boards, and knives to simplify the process of preparing cancer-fighting dishes. Simplify your cooking so that the enjoyment of preparing wholesome meals may take centre stage.

8. Conscious Cooking Setting:
Beyond actual food and equipment, design a conscious kitchen environment. Making food can become a healing ritual if it is done with focus, appreciation, and a positive outlook. This emotional component of cooking adds to the comprehensive character of cancer-prevention meals.

Equipped with these necessary kitchen tools, you're not simply creating meals, but also building a gourmet sanctuary where the combination of flavours becomes a potent weapon against cancer.

This chapter serves as your guide, teaching you the craft of choosing, chopping, and mixing these necessities into a harmonious blend of tastes and well-being. Greetings from the kitchen, where each ingredient serves as a tool to paint a picture of health and each recipe showcases the power of a well-fed body and mind.

10 Quick and Easy Breakfast Recipes

1. Berry and Greek Yogurt Parfait:

Ingredients:
   - 1 cup Greek yogurt
   - 1/2 cup granola
   - 1/2 cup mixed berries (strawberries, blueberries, raspberries)
   - 1 tablespoon honey (optional)

Preparation:
   1. In a glass or a bowl, start with a layer of Greek yogurt.
   2. Add a layer of granola on top of the yogurt.
   3. Place a handful of mixed berries over the granola layer.
   4. Repeat the layers until you reach the top, finishing with a drizzle of honey if desired.

5. Serve immediately and enjoy the vibrant flavors and textures.

2. Avocado Toast with Poached Egg:

Ingredients:
- 1 slice whole-grain bread
- 1/2 ripe avocado
- 1 large egg
- Salt and pepper to taste
- Optional toppings: red pepper flakes, cherry tomatoes

Preparation:
1. Toast the whole-grain bread to your desired level of crispiness.
2. While the bread is toasting, mash the ripe avocado and spread it evenly over the toasted bread.
3. In a small saucepan, bring water to a gentle simmer. Add a splash of vinegar.

4. Crack the egg into a small bowl and gently slide it into the simmering water. Poach the egg for about 3-4 minutes for a runny yolk.

5. Using a slotted spoon, carefully remove the poached egg from the water and place it on top of the avocado toast.

6. Season with salt and pepper to taste. Add optional toppings like red pepper flakes or sliced cherry tomatoes.

7. Serve immediately, and enjoy a satisfying breakfast rich in healthy fats and protein.

3. Oatmeal with Nut Butter and Banana Slices:

Ingredients:
- 1/2 cup rolled oats
- 1 cup milk (dairy or plant-based)
- 1 tablespoon nut butter (almond, peanut, or your choice)
- 1 ripe banana, sliced

- 1 tablespoon honey or maple syrup (optional)
- Nuts or seeds for garnish (optional)

Preparation:

1. In a small saucepan, combine rolled oats and milk. Bring to a gentle simmer over medium heat.
2. Stir the oats frequently until they reach your desired consistency.
3. Once cooked, transfer the oatmeal to a bowl.
4. Swirl in the nut butter, add banana slices, and drizzle with honey or maple syrup if desired.
5. Garnish with nuts or seeds for added crunch.
6. Serve warm and enjoy a comforting and nutrient-packed breakfast.

4. Vegetable Omelette with Whole Grain Toast:

Ingredients:
- 2 large eggs
- Salt and pepper to taste
- 1 tablespoon olive oil
- 1/4 cup diced bell peppers
- 1/4 cup diced tomatoes
- 1/4 cup diced onions
- 1/4 cup shredded cheese (optional)
- 1 slice whole-grain bread, toasted

Preparation:
1. Crack the eggs into a bowl, season with salt and pepper, and whisk until well combined.
2. Heat olive oil in a non-stick skillet over medium heat.
3. Add diced bell peppers, tomatoes, and onions to the skillet. Sauté until the vegetables are tender.

4. Pour the whisked eggs over the sautéed vegetables, tilting the pan to spread them evenly.

5. Allow the eggs to set around the edges, then gently lift and fold the omelette in half.

6. If desired, sprinkle shredded cheese over the omelette and let it melt.

7. Slide the omelette onto a plate and serve with a slice of whole-grain toast.

5. Chia Seed Pudding with Berries:

Ingredients:
  - 3 tablespoons chia seeds
  - 1 cup milk (dairy or plant-based)
  - 1/2 teaspoon vanilla extract
  - 1 tablespoon honey or maple syrup
  - Mixed berries for topping

Preparation:

1. In a bowl, combine chia seeds, milk, vanilla extract, and honey or maple syrup. Stir well.

2. Let the mixture sit for 5 minutes, then stir again to prevent clumping. Cover and refrigerate for at least 2 hours or overnight.

3. Before serving, give the chia pudding a good stir. Adjust the sweetness if needed.

4. Top with a generous handful of mixed berries.

5. Serve chilled and savor the creamy texture and burst of flavors.

6. Smoothie Bowl with Spinach and Tropical Fruits:

Ingredients:

- 1 cup frozen tropical fruits (pineapple, mango, banana)
- 1/2 cup fresh spinach leaves

- 1/2 cup almond milk (or any preferred milk)
- Toppings: granola, sliced banana, shredded coconut, chia seeds

Preparation:
1. In a blender, combine frozen tropical fruits, fresh spinach, and almond milk.
2. Blend until smooth, adding more liquid if necessary to reach a thick but pourable consistency.
3. Pour the smoothie into a bowl.
4. Top with granola, sliced banana, shredded coconut, and a sprinkle of chia seeds.
5. Customize with additional toppings if desired.
6. Enjoy a refreshing and nutrient-packed smoothie bowl to kickstart your morning.

7. Quinoa Breakfast Bowl:

Ingredients:
- 1/2 cup cooked quinoa
- 1/2 cup sliced strawberries
- 1/4 cup blueberries
- 2 tablespoons chopped nuts (almonds, walnuts, or your choice)
- 1 tablespoon honey or maple syrup
- Greek yogurt for topping

Preparation:
1. In a bowl, layer cooked quinoa as the base.
2. Top with sliced strawberries, blueberries, and chopped nuts.
3. Drizzle honey or maple syrup over the bowl for sweetness.
4. Add a dollop of Greek yogurt on top.
5. Mix all the ingredients before enjoying a protein-packed and satisfying breakfast bowl.

Ingredients:
- 1 cup whole wheat flour
- 1 tablespoon baking powder
- 1 tablespoon sugar
- 1 cup milk (dairy or plant-based)
- 1 large egg
- 1 tablespoon melted butter
- Blueberry Compote: 1 cup blueberries, 2 tablespoons maple syrup, 1 teaspoon lemon juice

Preparation:

For Pancakes:

1. In a bowl, whisk together whole wheat flour, baking powder, and sugar.

2. In a separate bowl, whisk together milk, egg, and melted butter.

3. Combine wet and dry ingredients until just mixed.

4. Heat a griddle or non-stick skillet over medium heat.

5. Pour 1/4 cup batter for each pancake onto the griddle. Cook until bubbles form, then flip and cook until golden brown.

For Blueberry Compote:

1. In a saucepan, combine blueberries, maple syrup, and lemon juice.

2. Simmer over medium heat until the blueberries burst and the mixture thickens slightly.

3. Serve the pancakes topped with warm blueberry compote. Enjoy a delightful and wholesome breakfast!

9. Yogurt and Fruit Smoothie:

Ingredients:

- 1 cup yogurt (Greek or regular, plain or flavored)

- 1/2 cup mixed fruits (berries, banana, mango)

- 1 handful spinach leaves
- 1/2 cup almond milk (or any preferred milk)
- 1 tablespoon chia seeds (optional)
- Honey or maple syrup for sweetness (optional)

Preparation:
1. In a blender, combine yogurt, mixed fruits, spinach leaves, almond milk, and chia seeds.
2. Blend until smooth, adjusting the sweetness with honey or maple syrup if needed.
3. Pour into a glass or bowl.
4. Garnish with additional fruit slices or a sprinkle of chia seeds.
5. Sip and savor the refreshing and nutrient-rich smoothie.

10. Egg Muffins with Spinach and Feta:

Ingredients:
- 4 large eggs
- 1/4 cup milk
- Salt and pepper to taste
- 1 cup fresh spinach, chopped
- 1/4 cup feta cheese, crumbled
- 1/4 cup cherry tomatoes, halved
- Cooking spray or olive oil for greasing

Preparation:
1. Preheat the oven to 375°F (190°C). Grease a muffin tin with cooking spray or olive oil.

2. In a bowl, whisk together eggs, milk, salt, and pepper.

3. Stir in chopped spinach, crumbled feta, and cherry tomatoes.

4. Pour the mixture evenly into the muffin cups.

5. Bake for 20-25 minutes or until the egg muffins are set and slightly golden.

6. Allow them to cool for a few minutes before removing from the muffin tin.

10 Wholesome Lunch Ideas

1. Quinoa Salad with Chickpeas and Vegetables:

Ingredients:
- 1 cup quinoa, rinsed
- 2 cups water or vegetable broth
- 1 can (15 oz) chickpeas, drained and rinsed
- 1 cup cherry tomatoes, halved
- 1 cucumber, diced
- 1/2 red onion, finely chopped
- 1/4 cup feta cheese, crumbled
- Fresh parsley, chopped
- Olive oil, lemon juice, salt, and pepper for dressing

Preparation:

1. Cook quinoa according to package instructions, using water or vegetable broth for added flavor.

2. In a large bowl, combine cooked quinoa, chickpeas, cherry tomatoes, cucumber, red onion, and feta cheese.

3. In a small bowl, whisk together olive oil, lemon juice, salt, and pepper for the dressing.

4. Drizzle the dressing over the salad and toss until well combined.

5. Garnish with fresh parsley.

6. Serve chilled or at room temperature for a wholesome and satisfying lunch.

2. Grilled Chicken Wrap with Avocado and Hummus:

Ingredients:
- 1 boneless, skinless chicken breast
- 1 tablespoon olive oil

- 1 teaspoon cumin
- Salt and pepper to taste
- Whole grain wraps
- 1 ripe avocado, sliced
- 1/2 cup hummus
- Cherry tomatoes, lettuce, and cucumber for filling

Preparation:
1. Preheat the grill or a grill pan over medium-high heat.
2. Rub the chicken breast with olive oil, cumin, salt, and pepper.
3. Grill the chicken for 6-8 minutes per side or until fully cooked.
4. Slice the grilled chicken into strips.
5. Lay out the whole grain wraps and spread hummus over each one.
6. Arrange sliced avocado, grilled chicken, cherry tomatoes, lettuce, and cucumber down the center of each wrap.

7. Fold in the sides of the wrap and then roll it up tightly.

8. Slice in half if desired and serve as a wholesome and protein-packed lunch.

3. Mediterranean Chickpea Salad:

Ingredients:
- 2 cans (15 oz each) chickpeas, drained and rinsed
- 1 cup cherry tomatoes, halved
- 1 cucumber, diced
- 1/2 red onion, finely chopped
- 1 cup Kalamata olives, pitted and sliced
- 1 cup feta cheese, crumbled
- Fresh parsley, chopped
- 1/4 cup extra-virgin olive oil
- 2 tablespoons red wine vinegar
- 1 teaspoon dried oregano
- Salt and pepper to taste

Preparation:

1. In a large bowl, combine chickpeas, cherry tomatoes, cucumber, red onion, olives, and feta cheese.

2. In a small bowl, whisk together olive oil, red wine vinegar, dried oregano, salt, and pepper for the dressing.

3. Pour the dressing over the salad and toss gently to combine.

4. Garnish with fresh parsley.

5. Allow the salad to marinate for at least 30 minutes before serving for enhanced flavor.

6. Serve as a refreshing and protein-rich Mediterranean-inspired lunch.

4. Vegetarian Buddha Bowl:

Ingredients:
- 1 cup cooked quinoa
- 1 cup roasted sweet potatoes, cubed
- 1 cup sautéed kale or spinach
- 1/2 cup shredded carrots

- 1/2 cup edamame, shelled
- 1 avocado, sliced
- 1/4 cup hummus
- Sesame seeds and a drizzle of tahini for topping

Preparation:
1. Assemble the bowl with cooked quinoa as the base.
2. Arrange roasted sweet potatoes, sautéed kale or spinach, shredded carrots, edamame, and avocado in separate sections on top of the quinoa.
3. Add a dollop of hummus in one section of the bowl.
4. Drizzle tahini over the bowl and sprinkle sesame seeds for added crunch.
5. Mix the components together before enjoying a nutrient-packed and visually appealing Buddha Bowl.
6. Customize with your favorite sauces or additional toppings.

Ingredients:
- 4 bell peppers, halved and seeds removed
- 1 cup quinoa, cooked
- 2 cans (6 oz each) canned salmon, drained and flaked
- 1 cup cherry tomatoes, diced
- 1/2 cup red onion, finely chopped
- 1/4 cup fresh dill, chopped
- 1/4 cup feta cheese, crumbled
- Lemon wedges for serving
- Olive oil, salt, and pepper

Preparation:
1. Preheat the oven to 375°F (190°C).
2. In a bowl, combine cooked quinoa, flaked salmon, cherry tomatoes, red

onion, dill, feta cheese, a drizzle of olive oil, salt, and pepper.

3. Stuff each bell pepper half with the quinoa and salmon mixture.

4. Place the stuffed peppers in a baking dish.

5. Bake for 25-30 minutes or until the peppers are tender.

6. Serve with lemon wedges for a zesty touch.

6. Chickpea and Vegetable Stir-Fry:

Ingredients:
- 1 can (15 oz) chickpeas, drained and rinsed
- 2 cups broccoli florets
- 1 red bell pepper, sliced
- 1 carrot, julienned
- 1 zucchini, sliced
- 2 tablespoons soy sauce
- 1 tablespoon sesame oil

- 1 tablespoon ginger, minced
- 2 cloves garlic, minced
- Green onions and sesame seeds for garnish
- Cooked brown rice for serving

Preparation:

1. Heat sesame oil in a large skillet or wok over medium-high heat.

2. Add ginger and garlic, sauté for 1-2 minutes until fragrant.

3. Add broccoli, bell pepper, carrot, and zucchini to the skillet. Stir-fry for 5-7 minutes until the vegetables are tender-crisp.

4. Stir in chickpeas and soy sauce, cooking for an additional 2-3 minutes.

5. Serve the stir-fry over cooked brown rice.

6. Garnish with sliced green onions and sesame seeds before serving.

7. Caprese Quinoa Bowl:

Ingredients:
- 1 cup quinoa, cooked
- 1 cup cherry tomatoes, halved
- 1 cup fresh mozzarella balls
- 1 cup fresh basil leaves
- 2 tablespoons balsamic glaze
- 2 tablespoons extra-virgin olive oil
- Salt and pepper to taste

Preparation:
1. In a bowl, combine cooked quinoa, cherry tomatoes, fresh mozzarella balls, and fresh basil leaves.
2. Drizzle with balsamic glaze and extra-virgin olive oil.
3. Season with salt and pepper to taste.
4. Toss the ingredients gently until well combined.

5. Serve at room temperature for a refreshing and satisfying Caprese-inspired quinoa bowl.

8. Sweet Potato and Black Bean Quesadillas:

Ingredients:
- 2 medium sweet potatoes, peeled and diced
- 1 can (15 oz) black beans, drained and rinsed
- 1 teaspoon cumin
- 1 teaspoon chili powder
- 1/2 teaspoon paprika
- Salt and pepper to taste
- 4 whole wheat or corn tortillas
- 1 cup shredded cheese (cheddar or Mexican blend)
- Fresh cilantro and lime wedges for serving

Preparation:

1. Steam or boil the diced sweet potatoes until tender. Mash them in a bowl.

2. In a skillet, combine mashed sweet potatoes, black beans, cumin, chili powder, paprika, salt, and pepper. Cook until heated through.

3. Lay out the tortillas and spread the sweet potato and black bean mixture on half of each tortilla.

4. Sprinkle shredded cheese over the mixture and fold the tortillas in half.

5. Heat a skillet over medium heat and cook each quesadilla for 2-3 minutes on each side until the cheese is melted and the tortilla is golden brown.

6. Serve with fresh cilantro and lime wedges on the side.

9. Veggie-Packed Quinoa Bowl with Tahini Dressing:

Ingredients:

- 1 cup quinoa, cooked
- 1 cup cherry tomatoes, halved
- 1 cucumber, diced
- 1 bell pepper, thinly sliced
- 1/2 red onion, finely chopped
- 1 cup cooked chickpeas
- 1/4 cup crumbled feta cheese
- Fresh parsley, chopped
- For Tahini Dressing:
  - 3 tablespoons tahini
  - 2 tablespoons lemon juice
  - 1 tablespoon olive oil
  - 1 clove garlic, minced
  - Salt and pepper to taste
  - Water to thin, if necessary

Preparation:

1. In a bowl, combine cooked quinoa, cherry tomatoes, cucumber, bell pepper, red onion, chickpeas, and feta cheese.

2. In a small bowl, whisk together tahini, lemon juice, olive oil, minced garlic, salt, and pepper. Add water to thin the dressing if necessary.

3. Drizzle the tahini dressing over the quinoa bowl and toss until well coated.

4. Garnish with fresh parsley.

5. Serve at room temperature for a vibrant and nutrient-packed lunch.

10. Lentil and Vegetable Curry:

Ingredients:
- 1 cup dried lentils, rinsed and drained
- 1 tablespoon coconut oil
- 1 onion, diced
- 2 cloves garlic, minced
- 1 tablespoon curry powder
- 1 teaspoon ground cumin
- 1 teaspoon ground coriander
- 1 can (14 oz) diced tomatoes
- 1 can (14 oz) coconut milk

- 2 cups mixed vegetables (such as broccoli, carrots, bell peppers)
- Salt and pepper to taste
- Fresh cilantro for garnish
- Cooked brown rice for serving

Preparation:
1. In a large pot, heat coconut oil over medium heat. Add diced onion and cook until softened.
2. Add minced garlic, curry powder, ground cumin, and ground coriander. Stir and cook for 1-2 minutes until fragrant.
3. Add rinsed lentils, diced tomatoes, coconut milk, and mixed vegetables to the pot.
4. Bring the mixture to a simmer, then reduce the heat and let it cook until the lentils and vegetables are tender.
5. Season with salt and pepper to taste.

6. Serve the lentil and vegetable curry over cooked brown rice, garnished with fresh cilantro.

Nutrient-Packed Dinner Delights

Dinner is not just a meal; it's an opportunity to nourish the body with a symphony of flavors and essential nutrients. These nutrient-packed dinner delights not only tantalize the taste buds but also provide a well-rounded array of vitamins, minerals, and wholesome goodness. Let's explore a culinary journey that celebrates health and flavor in every bite.

1. Salmon and Quinoa Power Bowl:

Ingredients:

- 2 salmon fillets
- 1 cup quinoa, cooked
- 1 cup broccoli florets, steamed
- 1/2 cup cherry tomatoes, halved
- 1/4 cup red onion, finely chopped
- 1/4 cup feta cheese, crumbled
- Lemon wedges for serving
- Olive oil, salt, and pepper

Preparation:

1. Season salmon fillets with olive oil, salt, and pepper. Bake or grill until cooked through.

2. In a bowl, assemble cooked quinoa, steamed broccoli, cherry tomatoes, red onion, and crumbled feta.

3. Top with the cooked salmon fillets.

4. Serve with lemon wedges for a burst of freshness.

2. Vegetarian Stuffed Bell Peppers:

Ingredients:

- 4 bell peppers, halved and seeds removed
- 1 cup quinoa, cooked
- 1 can (15 oz) black beans, drained and rinsed
- 1 cup corn kernels
- 1 cup cherry tomatoes, diced
- 1/2 cup red onion, finely chopped
- 1 cup spinach, chopped
- 1 teaspoon cumin
- 1 teaspoon chili powder
- Salt and pepper to taste
- Shredded cheese for topping

Preparation:

1. Preheat the oven to 375°F (190°C).

2. In a bowl, mix cooked quinoa, black beans, corn, cherry tomatoes, red onion, spinach, cumin, chili powder, salt, and pepper.

3. Stuff each bell pepper half with the quinoa mixture.

4. Top with shredded cheese.

5. Bake for 25-30 minutes or until the peppers are tender.

3. Chickpea and Vegetable Stir-Fry:

Ingredients:
- 1 can (15 oz) chickpeas, drained and rinsed
- 2 cups broccoli florets
- 1 bell pepper, sliced
- 1 carrot, julienned
- 1 zucchini, sliced
- 2 tablespoons soy sauce
- 1 tablespoon sesame oil
- 1 tablespoon ginger, minced
- 2 cloves garlic, minced
- Green onions and sesame seeds for garnish
- Cooked brown rice for serving

Preparation:

1. Heat sesame oil in a large skillet or wok over medium-high heat.

2. Add ginger and garlic, sauté for 1-2 minutes until fragrant.

3. Add broccoli, bell pepper, carrot, and zucchini to the skillet. Stir-fry for 5-7 minutes until the vegetables are tender-crisp.

4. Stir in chickpeas and soy sauce, cooking for an additional 2-3 minutes.

5. Serve the stir-fry over cooked brown rice.

6. Garnish with sliced green onions and sesame seeds.

4. Mediterranean Grilled Chicken Salad:

Ingredients:
- 2 boneless, skinless chicken breasts
- 1 teaspoon dried oregano

- 1 teaspoon garlic powder
- Salt and pepper to taste
- 1 cup cherry tomatoes, halved
- 1 cucumber, diced
- 1/2 red onion, thinly sliced
- 1/4 cup Kalamata olives, pitted and sliced
- 1/4 cup feta cheese, crumbled
- Fresh parsley, chopped
- Olive oil and lemon juice for dressing

Preparation:

1. Season chicken breasts with dried oregano, garlic powder, salt, and pepper.

2. Grill the chicken until fully cooked, then slice into strips.

3. In a large bowl, combine cherry tomatoes, cucumber, red onion, olives, and feta cheese.

4. Add the grilled chicken strips on top.

5. Drizzle with olive oil and lemon juice for a light and flavorful dressing.

6. Garnish with fresh parsley.

5. Sweet Potato and Chickpea Curry:

Ingredients:
- 2 large sweet potatoes, peeled and diced
- 1 can (15 oz) chickpeas, drained and rinsed
- 1 onion, finely chopped
- 2 cloves garlic, minced
- 1 tablespoon ginger, grated
- 1 can (14 oz) diced tomatoes
- 1 can (14 oz) coconut milk
- 2 tablespoons curry powder
- 1 teaspoon ground cumin
- 1 teaspoon ground coriander
- 1/2 teaspoon turmeric
- Salt and pepper to taste
- Fresh cilantro for garnish
- Cooked brown rice for serving

Preparation:

1. In a large pot, sauté the chopped onion, garlic, and grated ginger until softened.

2. Add the diced sweet potatoes and chickpeas to the pot.

3. Sprinkle in the curry powder, ground cumin, ground coriander, turmeric, salt, and pepper. Stir to coat the ingredients with the spices.

4. Pour in the diced tomatoes and coconut milk. Stir well.

5. Bring the mixture to a boil, then reduce the heat and let it simmer until the sweet potatoes are tender.

6. Adjust the seasoning if necessary.

7. Serve the sweet potato and chickpea curry over cooked brown rice.

8. Garnish with fresh cilantro for a burst of freshness.

Ingredients:
- 1 cup dried green or brown lentils, rinsed
- 1 onion, finely chopped
- 2 carrots, diced
- 2 celery stalks, chopped
- 3 cloves garlic, minced
- 1 can (14 oz) diced tomatoes
- 6 cups vegetable broth
- 1 teaspoon ground cumin
- 1 teaspoon smoked paprika
- 1/2 teaspoon turmeric
- Salt and pepper to taste
- Fresh parsley for garnish
- Lemon wedges for serving

Preparation:

1. In a large pot, sauté the chopped onion, carrots, celery, and garlic until softened.

2. Add lentils, diced tomatoes, vegetable broth, ground cumin, smoked paprika, turmeric, salt, and pepper to the pot.

3. Bring the soup to a boil, then reduce the heat and let it simmer until the lentils are tender.

4. Adjust the seasoning if needed.

5. Serve the lentil soup hot, garnished with fresh parsley, and accompanied by lemon wedges for a citrusy kick.

7. Grilled Vegetable Quinoa Bowl:

Ingredients:
- 1 cup quinoa, cooked
- 1 zucchini, sliced
- 1 eggplant, sliced
- 1 bell pepper, sliced
- 1 cup cherry tomatoes

- 1/4 cup feta cheese, crumbled
- 2 tablespoons balsamic glaze
- Olive oil, salt, and pepper

Preparation:
1. Preheat the grill or a grill pan over medium-high heat.
2. Brush zucchini, eggplant, bell pepper, and cherry tomatoes with olive oil. Season with salt and pepper.
3. Grill the vegetables until they have nice grill marks and are cooked through.
4. In a bowl, assemble cooked quinoa, grilled vegetables, and crumbled feta cheese.
5. Drizzle with balsamic glaze.
6. Toss gently to combine and serve for a satisfying and nutritious dinner.

8. Teriyaki Tofu Stir-Fry:

Ingredients:

- 1 block firm tofu, pressed and cubed
- 2 tablespoons soy sauce
- 2 tablespoons teriyaki sauce
- 1 tablespoon sesame oil
- 1 tablespoon ginger, minced
- 2 cloves garlic, minced
- 1 broccoli crown, florets separated
- 1 bell pepper, sliced
- 1 carrot, julienned
- 1 cup snap peas, ends trimmed
- 2 green onions, sliced
- Sesame seeds for garnish
- Cooked brown rice or quinoa for serving

Preparation:

1. In a bowl, marinate cubed tofu in soy sauce and teriyaki sauce for 15-20 minutes.

2. In a large skillet or wok, heat sesame oil over medium-high heat.

3. Add marinated tofu and cook until golden brown on all sides. Remove from the skillet and set aside.

4. In the same skillet, add ginger and garlic, sauté for 1-2 minutes until fragrant.

5. Add broccoli, bell pepper, carrot, and snap peas. Stir-fry until the vegetables are crisp-tender.

6. Return the cooked tofu to the skillet and add sliced green onions. Toss everything together.

7. Serve the teriyaki tofu stir-fry over cooked brown rice or quinoa.

8. Garnish with sesame seeds for added crunch.

9. Chickpea and Spinach Curry:

Ingredients:
- 2 cans (15 oz each) chickpeas, drained and rinsed
- 1 tablespoon coconut oil

- 1 large onion, finely chopped
- 3 cloves garlic, minced
- 1 tablespoon curry powder
- 1 teaspoon ground cumin
- 1 teaspoon ground coriander
- 1 teaspoon turmeric
- 1 can (14 oz) diced tomatoes
- 1 can (14 oz) coconut milk
- 4 cups fresh spinach
- Salt and pepper to taste
- Fresh cilantro for garnish
- Cooked basmati rice for serving

Preparation:

1. In a large pot, heat coconut oil over medium heat. Add chopped onion and cook until softened.

2. Add minced garlic, curry powder, ground cumin, ground coriander, and turmeric. Stir for 1-2 minutes until fragrant.

3. Pour in diced tomatoes, coconut milk, and drained chickpeas. Simmer for 15-20 minutes.

4. Stir in fresh spinach and cook until wilted.

5. Season with salt and pepper to taste.

6. Serve the chickpea and spinach curry over cooked basmati rice.

7. Garnish with fresh cilantro.

10. Baked Stuffed Bell Peppers with Turkey and Quinoa:

Ingredients:
- 4 large bell peppers, halved and seeds removed
- 1 cup quinoa, cooked
- 1 lb ground turkey
- 1 onion, finely chopped
- 2 cloves garlic, minced
- 1 can (14 oz) diced tomatoes, drained
- 1 teaspoon Italian seasoning

- Salt and pepper to taste
- 1 cup shredded mozzarella cheese
- Fresh basil for garnish

Preparation:

1. Preheat the oven to 375°F (190°C).

2. In a skillet, cook ground turkey until browned. Add chopped onion and garlic, sauté until softened.

3. Stir in cooked quinoa, diced tomatoes, Italian seasoning, salt, and pepper.

4. Stuff each bell pepper half with the turkey and quinoa mixture.

5. Top with shredded mozzarella cheese.

6. Bake for 25-30 minutes or until the peppers are tender and the cheese is melted and bubbly.

7. Garnish with fresh basil before serving.

Snack Time Goodies for a Healthy Boost

Snack time doesn't have to be synonymous with processed treats and empty calories. Elevate your snack game with these 10 goodies that not only satisfy your cravings but also provide a nutritious boost to fuel your day.

1. Greek Yogurt Parfait:

Ingredients:
- 1 cup Greek yogurt (plain or flavored)
- 1/2 cup granola
- 1/2 cup mixed berries
- Drizzle of honey

Preparation:
Layer Greek yogurt with granola and mixed berries in a glass or bowl. Drizzle

with honey for added sweetness. This parfait delivers a protein punch from the yogurt, fiber from the granola, and antioxidants from the berries.

2. Almond Butter and Banana Rice Cakes:

Ingredients:
- Rice cakes
- Almond butter
- Banana, sliced

Preparation:
Spread almond butter on rice cakes and top with banana slices. This snack combines the healthy fats of almond butter, the crunch of rice cakes, and the potassium-rich goodness of bananas.

3. Veggie Sticks with Hummus:

Ingredients:

- Carrot sticks
- Cucumber slices
- Cherry tomatoes
- Hummus

Preparation:

Dip colorful veggie sticks in hummus for a refreshing and satisfying snack. The vegetables offer vitamins and minerals, while hummus provides protein and a flavorful kick.

4. Chia Seed Pudding:

Ingredients:
- 3 tablespoons chia seeds
- 1 cup almond milk
- 1 teaspoon vanilla extract
- Fresh fruit for topping

Preparation:

Mix chia seeds with almond milk and vanilla extract. Let it sit in the refrigerator for a few hours or overnight until it forms a pudding-like consistency. Top with fresh fruit for a nutritious and customizable snack.

5. Edamame with Sea Salt:

Ingredients:
- Edamame (steamed or boiled)
- Sea salt

Preparation:
Sprinkle steamed edamame with a pinch of sea salt for a protein-packed snack rich in fiber and essential amino acids.

6. Trail Mix with Nuts and Dried Fruit:

Ingredients:

- Mixed nuts (almonds, walnuts, cashews)
- Dried fruits (raisins, apricots, cranberries)
- Dark chocolate chips (optional)

Preparation:
Create a custom trail mix by combining assorted nuts, dried fruits, and dark chocolate chips for a delightful blend of textures and flavors.

7. Avocado Toast:

Ingredients:
- Whole-grain bread
- Ripe avocado
- Cherry tomatoes, sliced
- Sprinkle of black sesame seeds

Preparation:

Mash ripe avocado on whole-grain toast and top with sliced cherry tomatoes and a sprinkle of black sesame seeds. This snack offers healthy fats, fiber, and a satisfying crunch.

8. Cottage Cheese and Pineapple Cups:

Ingredients:
- Cottage cheese
- Fresh pineapple chunks

Preparation:
Serve cottage cheese in small cups and top with fresh pineapple chunks. This combination provides protein, vitamins, and a tropical twist.

9. Roasted Chickpeas:

Ingredients:
- Canned chickpeas, drained and rinsed

- Olive oil
- Paprika, cumin, garlic powder (or preferred spices)

Preparation:
Toss chickpeas with olive oil and spices, then roast in the oven until crispy. Roasted chickpeas are a crunchy and protein-rich snack.

10. Apple Slices with Nut Butter:

Ingredients:
- Apple slices
- Nut butter (peanut, almond, or cashew)

Preparation:
Spread your favorite nut butter on apple slices for a delicious combination of natural sweetness, fiber, and healthy fats.

Desserts That Satisfy Sweet Cravings Without Compromising Health

Indulging in desserts doesn't have to mean sacrificing your commitment to a healthy lifestyle. These 10 delectable treats are not only irresistibly sweet but also boast nutritional benefits, making them the perfect guilt-free indulgence for those with a sweet tooth.

1. Chia Seed Pudding with Fresh Fruit:

Ingredients:
- 3 tablespoons chia seeds
- 1 cup almond milk
- 1 teaspoon vanilla extract
- Fresh fruit for topping

Preparation:

Combine chia seeds, almond milk, and vanilla extract. Allow it to set in the refrigerator until it reaches a pudding-like consistency. Top with your favorite fresh fruit for added natural sweetness and vitamins.

2. Dark Chocolate-Dipped Strawberries:

Ingredients:
- Fresh strawberries
- Dark chocolate (70% cocoa or higher)

Preparation:
Melt dark chocolate and dip fresh strawberries for a delightful combination of antioxidants from the chocolate and vitamin C from the strawberries.

3. Baked Apples with Cinnamon:

Ingredients:

- Apples, cored and sliced
- Cinnamon
- Nutmeg (optional)
- Greek yogurt for serving

Preparation:

Arrange apple slices in a baking dish, sprinkle with cinnamon (and nutmeg if desired), and bake until tender. Serve with a dollop of Greek yogurt for a comforting and nutritious dessert.

4. Frozen Banana Bites:

Ingredients:
- Bananas, sliced
- Almond butter
- Dark chocolate

Preparation:

Spread almond butter on banana slices, then dip in melted dark chocolate. Freeze

until solid for a satisfying and
portion-controlled sweet treat.

5. Avocado Chocolate Mousse:

Ingredients:
- Ripe avocados
- Cocoa powder
- Maple syrup or honey
- Vanilla extract

Preparation:
Blend ripe avocados with cocoa powder,
sweeten with maple syrup or honey, and
add a splash of vanilla extract. The result
is a creamy chocolate mousse rich in
healthy fats.

6. Yogurt Parfait with Nuts and Berries:

Ingredients:
- Greek yogurt (plain or flavored)

- Mixed berries
- Nuts (almonds, walnuts)

Preparation:
Layer Greek yogurt with fresh berries and nuts for a dessert that's high in protein, fiber, and antioxidants.

7. Coconut and Almond Energy Balls:

Ingredients:
- Dates, pitted
- Almonds
- Shredded coconut
- Cocoa powder

Preparation:
Blend dates, almonds, shredded coconut, and cocoa powder into energy balls. These bites are not only sweet but also packed with natural sugars and healthy fats.

8. Baked Peaches with Cinnamon:

Ingredients:
- Peaches, halved and pitted
- Cinnamon
- Honey (optional)

Preparation:
Place peach halves on a baking sheet, sprinkle with cinnamon, and bake until tender. Drizzle with honey if desired for a warm and satisfying dessert.

9. Quinoa Pudding with Berries:

Ingredients:
- Cooked quinoa
- Almond milk
- Vanilla extract
- Mixed berrics

Preparation:

Combine cooked quinoa with almond milk and vanilla extract. Top with mixed berries for a wholesome and satisfying pudding.

10. Cinnamon Roasted Sweet Potatoes:

Ingredients:
- Sweet potatoes, peeled and diced
- Cinnamon
- Maple syrup

Preparation:

Toss sweet potatoes with cinnamon and a drizzle of maple syrup before roasting. These sweet and spiced sweet potatoes make for a nutritious and delightful dessert alternative.

These desserts are proof that you can indulge your sweet cravings while still nourishing your body with wholesome ingredients. Enjoy these treats as part of a balanced diet, and savor the satisfaction of a healthier approach to dessert time.

Beverages for Hydration and Nutritional Support

Staying hydrated is crucial for overall well-being, and incorporating nutrient-rich beverages into your routine ensures not only hydration but also a boost of essential vitamins and minerals. Explore these beverages that not only quench your thirst but also contribute to your nutritional needs.

1. Green Tea:

Benefits:

- Rich in antioxidants, particularly catechins.

- Supports metabolism and may aid in weight management.

- Contains L-theanine for a calming effect.

Preparation:

Brew green tea leaves or use green tea bags. Customize with lemon or a touch of honey for added flavor.

2. Infused Water:

Benefits:

- Enhances hydration with a burst of natural flavors.

- Provides a low-calorie option for those watching their calorie intake.

- Can be customized with various fruits and herbs.

Preparation:
Combine water with slices of citrus fruits, berries, cucumber, or mint leaves. Allow it to infuse in the refrigerator for a refreshing drink.

3. Vegetable Juice:

Benefits:
- Packed with vitamins and minerals from various vegetables.
- Offers a convenient way to increase vegetable intake.
- May support immune function and digestion.

Preparation:
Juice a mix of vegetables like carrots, celery, kale, and tomatoes. Add a dash of lemon juice for brightness.

4. Coconut Water:

Benefits:
- Naturally hydrating with electrolytes.
- Low in calories and sugar.
- Contains potassium, magnesium, and calcium.

Consumption:
Enjoy coconut water straight from the coconut or opt for packaged versions without added sugars.

5. Smoothies:

Benefits:
- Versatile and can be tailored to individual nutritional needs.
- Offers a convenient way to include fruits, vegetables, and protein.
- Provides a delicious and satisfying beverage.

Preparation:
Blend together fruits, leafy greens, yogurt or milk, and a protein source like nut butter or protein powder.

6. Herbal Tea:

Benefits:
- Caffeine-free options for those looking to reduce caffeine intake.
- Various herbal teas have unique health benefits (e.g., chamomile for relaxation, peppermint for digestion).
- Hydrating and comforting.

Varieties:
Explore chamomile, peppermint, hibiscus, or ginger tea for different flavors and potential health benefits.

7. Kombucha:

Benefits:

- A fermented beverage rich in probiotics.
- Supports gut health and digestion.
- Contains antioxidants.

Selection:

Choose unsweetened or lightly sweetened varieties to minimize added sugars. Flavors range from fruity to spicy.

8. Golden Milk (Turmeric Latte):

Benefits:

- Features anti-inflammatory properties from turmeric.
- Often includes other spices like ginger and cinnamon for added health benefits.
- Provides a soothing and warm beverage option.

Preparation:
Combine turmeric, ginger, cinnamon, and black pepper with milk (dairy or plant-based) and sweeten with honey or maple syrup.

9. Protein Shakes:

Benefits:
- Ideal for post-workout recovery.
- Supports muscle repair and growth.
- Convenient way to increase protein intake.

Ingredients:
Blend together protein powder, milk or a dairy-free alternative, fruits, and a spoonful of nut butter for a satisfying protein shake.

10. Homemade Electrolyte Drink:

Benefits:
- Replenishes electrolytes lost through sweating.
- Suitable for those engaging in physical activity or needing rehydration.
- Customizable and cost-effective.

Ingredients:
Mix water with a pinch of salt, a squeeze of citrus juice, and a touch of honey or maple syrup for natural sweetness.

Incorporating these beverages into your daily routine not only helps meet your hydration needs but also provides a nutritional boost. Experiment with different options to find the flavors and combinations that suit your preferences and health goals. Remember that moderation and variety are key for a well-balanced approach to beverage consumption.

30 Day Meal Plan

WEEK 1

Note: It's essential to consult with a healthcare professional or a registered dietitian to tailor any dietary plan to individual needs, especially during cancer treatment. This meal plan is a general guide and may need adjustments based on specific requirements.

Day 1:

Breakfast:
- Quinoa Breakfast Bowl with Berries and Almonds
- Green Tea

Lunch:
- Grilled Chicken Salad with Mixed Greens, Cherry Tomatoes, and Avocado

- Whole Grain Roll
- Lemon Water

Snack:
- Greek Yogurt Parfait with Mixed Berries and Chia Seeds

Dinner:
- Baked Salmon with Lemon and Dill
- Steamed Broccoli and Quinoa
- Herbal Tea

Day 2:

Breakfast:
- Oatmeal with Sliced Banana and Walnuts
- Green Smoothie (Spinach, Banana, Greek Yogurt, Almond Milk)

Lunch:
- Lentil and Vegetable Soup

- Whole Grain Crackers
- Infused Water with Cucumber and Mint

Snack:
- Fresh Fruit Salad with a Drizzle of
Honey

Dinner:
- Grilled Vegetable Stir-Fry with Tofu
- Brown Rice
- Turmeric Ginger Tea

Day 3:

Breakfast:
- Whole Grain Toast with Avocado and
Poached Egg
- Berry Smoothie (Blueberries,
Strawberries, Almond Milk)

Lunch:

- Chickpea and Spinach Salad with Lemon
Vinaigrette
- Quinoa Pilaf
- Coconut Water

Snack:
- Handful of Almonds and Dried Apricots

Dinner:
- Baked Chicken Breast with Herbs
- Sweet Potato Mash
- Steamed Asparagus
- Chamomile Tea

Day 4:

Breakfast:
- Greek Yogurt and Berry Smoothie Bowl
- Green Tea with Lemon

Lunch:

- Quinoa and Black Bean Stuffed Bell
Peppers
- Mixed Greens Salad
- Lemon Water

Snack:
- Hummus with Veggie Sticks (Carrots,
Cucumber, Bell Peppers)

Dinner:
- Shrimp and Vegetable Stir-Fry
- Brown Rice
- Herbal Infusion (Peppermint or Ginger)

Day 5:

Breakfast:
- Chia Seed Pudding with Mango and
Pistachios
- Turmeric Latte (Golden Milk)

Lunch:

- Mediterranean Grilled Chicken Salad
- Whole Grain Pita Bread
- Infused Water with Citrus Slices

Snack:
- Cottage Cheese with Pineapple Chunks

Dinner:
- Quinoa and Vegetable Buddha Bowl
- Tahini Dressing
- Herbal Tea Blend

Day 6:

Breakfast:
- Whole Grain Pancakes with Berries and Greek Yogurt
- Green Smoothie (Kale, Pineapple, Coconut Water)

Lunch:
- Tomato Basil Chickpea Pasta

- Mixed Greens Salad
- Lemon Water with Mint

Snack:
- Apple Slices with Almond Butter

Dinner:
- Baked Cod with Herbed Quinoa
- Roasted Brussels Sprouts
- Detoxifying Green Tea

Day 7:

Breakfast:
- Berry and Spinach Smoothie Bowl
- Matcha Green Tea Latte

Lunch:
- Lentil and Vegetable Wrap with Whole Grain Tortilla
- Sliced Watermelon
- Infused Water with Basil and Lime

Snack:
- Trail Mix (Nuts, Seeds, Dried Fruits)

Dinner:
- Vegetable Curry with Chickpeas
- Basmati Rice
- Herbal Infusion (Chamomile or Mint)

Remember to drink plenty of water throughout the day and adapt portion sizes based on individual needs and preferences.

WEEK 2

Day 1:

Breakfast:
- Overnight Chia Seed Pudding with Mixed Berries
- Green Tea with Lemon

Lunch:
- Quinoa Salad with Roasted Vegetables and Feta
- Whole Grain Roll
- Infused Water with Cucumber and Mint

Snack:
- Greek Yogurt with Honey and Almonds

Dinner:
- Grilled Salmon with Herb Quinoa
- Steamed Broccoli
- Herbal Tea (Chamomile or Peppermint)

Day 2:

Breakfast:
- Whole Grain Toast with Avocado and Poached Egg
- Berry Smoothie (Blueberries, Strawberries, Almond Milk)

Lunch:
- Lentil Soup with Whole Grain Crackers
- Mixed Greens Salad
- Lemon Water with Fresh Basil

Snack:
- Fresh Fruit Salad with a Drizzle of Honey

Dinner:
- Baked Chicken Thighs with Lemon and Rosemary
- Sweet Potato Mash
- Sautéed Spinach
- Turmeric Ginger Tea

Day 3:

Breakfast:
- Spinach and Feta Omelette
- Whole Grain English Muffin

- Green Tea with Mint

Lunch:
- Chickpea and Quinoa Stuffed Bell
Peppers
- Mixed Greens Salad
- Coconut Water

Snack:
- Hummus with Veggie Sticks (Carrots,
Cucumber, Bell Peppers)

Dinner:
- Shrimp and Vegetable Stir-Fry with
Brown Rice
- Steamed Asparagus
- Herbal Infusion (Lemon Balm or Ginger)

Day 4:

Breakfast:

- Whole Grain Pancakes with Berries and
Greek Yogurt
- Matcha Latte with Almond Milk

Lunch:
- Mediterranean Chickpea Salad with
Tzatziki Dressing
- Whole Grain Pita Bread
- Infused Water with Citrus Slices

Snack:
- Cottage Cheese with Pineapple Chunks

Dinner:
- Baked Cod with Quinoa Pilaf
- Roasted Brussels Sprouts
- Detoxifying Green Tea

Day 5:

Breakfast:
- Berry and Spinach Smoothie Bowl

- Turmeric Latte (Golden Milk)

Lunch:
- Quinoa and Black Bean Bowl with Avocado
- Lemon Water with Fresh Mint

Snack:
- Apple Slices with Almond Butter

Dinner:
- Vegetable Stir-Fry with Tofu and Brown Rice
- Herbal Tea Blend (Chamomile or Lavender)

Day 6:

Breakfast:
- Oatmeal with Sliced Banana and Walnuts

- Green Smoothie (Kale, Pineapple,
Coconut Water)

Lunch:
- Tomato Basil Chickpea Pasta
- Mixed Greens Salad
- Lemon Water with Rosemary

Snack:
- Trail Mix (Nuts, Seeds, Dried Fruits)

Dinner:
- Grilled Turkey Breast with Quinoa and
Vegetable Medley
- Herbal Infusion (Peppermint or
Echinacea)

Day 7:

Breakfast:
- Greek Yogurt Parfait with Mixed Berries
and Granola

- Matcha Green Tea

Lunch:
- Lentil and Vegetable Wrap with Whole Grain Tortilla
- Sliced Watermelon
- Infused Water with Basil and Lime

Snack:
- Almond Butter Banana Bites

Dinner:
- Vegetable Curry with Chickpeas and Basmati Rice
- Herbal Infusion (Chamomile or Lemongrass)

Remember to stay hydrated with water throughout the day and adjust portions based on individual needs and preferences.

WEEK 3

Day 1:

Breakfast:
- Quinoa Breakfast Bowl with Mixed Berries and Almonds
- Green Tea with Lemon

Lunch:
- Grilled Chicken Salad with Avocado, Cherry Tomatoes, and Balsamic Vinaigrette
- Whole Grain Roll
- Infused Water with Cucumber and Mint

Snack:
- Greek Yogurt Parfait with Chia Seeds and Fresh Berries

Dinner:
- Baked Salmon with Lemon and Dill

- Quinoa Pilaf
- Steamed Broccoli
- Herbal Tea (Chamomile or Ginger)

Day 2:

Breakfast:
- Overnight Chia Seed Pudding with Mango and Pistachios
- Turmeric Latte (Golden Milk)

Lunch:
- Lentil and Vegetable Soup
- Whole Grain Crackers
- Lemon Water with Fresh Basil

Snack:
- Fresh Fruit Salad with a Drizzle of Honey

Dinner:
- Grilled Shrimp and Vegetable Skewers

- Brown Rice
- Steamed Asparagus
- Herbal Infusion (Lemon Balm or Mint)

Day 3:

Breakfast:
- Spinach and Feta Omelette
- Whole Grain English Muffin
- Green Tea with Mint

Lunch:
- Chickpea and Spinach Salad with Lemon Tahini Dressing
- Quinoa Tabouli
- Coconut Water

Snack:
- Hummus with Veggie Sticks (Carrots, Cucumber, Bell Peppers)

Dinner:

- Teriyaki Tofu Stir-Fry with Brown Rice
- Sautéed Bok Choy
- Herbal Tea Blend (Chai or Lemongrass)

Day 4:

Breakfast:
- Whole Grain Pancakes with Mixed
Berries and Greek Yogurt
- Matcha Green Tea Latte

Lunch:
- Mediterranean Grilled Chicken Wrap
- Tzatziki Sauce
- Infused Water with Citrus Slices

Snack:
- Cottage Cheese with Pineapple Chunks

Dinner:
- Baked Cod with Quinoa and Vegetable
Medley

- Roasted Brussels Sprouts
- Detoxifying Green Tea

Day 5:

Breakfast:
- Berry and Spinach Smoothie Bowl
- Turmeric Ginger Tea

Lunch:
- Quinoa and Black Bean Stuffed Bell
Peppers
- Mixed Greens Salad
- Lemon Water with Fresh Mint

Snack:
- Apple Slices with Almond Butter

Dinner:
- Vegetable Stir-Fry with Tofu and Brown
Rice Noodles
- Ginger Sesame Sauce

- Herbal Infusion (Chamomile or Peppermint)

Day 6:

Breakfast:
- Oatmeal with Sliced Banana and Walnuts
- Green Smoothie (Kale, Pineapple, Coconut Water)

Lunch:
- Tomato Basil Chickpea Pasta
- Mixed Greens Salad
- Lemon Water with Rosemary

Snack:
- Trail Mix (Nuts, Seeds, Dried Fruits)

Dinner:
- Grilled Turkey Breast with Quinoa Pilaf
- Steamed Broccoli

- Herbal Infusion (Lavender or Echinacea)

Day 7:

Breakfast:
- Greek Yogurt Parfait with Mixed Berries and Granola
- Matcha Green Tea

Lunch:
- Lentil and Vegetable Wrap with Whole Grain Tortilla
- Sliced Watermelon
- Infused Water with Basil and Lime

Snack:
- Almond Butter Banana Bites

Dinner:
- Vegetable Curry with Chickpeas and Basmati Rice
- Sautéed Spinach

- Herbal Infusion (Chamomile or
Lemongrass)

Remember to stay hydrated with water
throughout the day and adjust portions
based on individual needs and
preferences.

WEEK 4

Day 1:

Breakfast:
- Quinoa Breakfast Bowl with Mixed
Berries and Almonds
- Green Tea with Lemon

Lunch:
- Grilled Chicken Salad with Avocado,
Cherry Tomatoes, and Balsamic
Vinaigrette
- Whole Grain Roll

- Infused Water with Cucumber and Mint

Snack:
- Greek Yogurt Parfait with Chia Seeds
and Fresh Berries

Dinner:
- Baked Salmon with Lemon and Dill
- Quinoa Pilaf
- Steamed Broccoli
- Herbal Tea (Chamomile or Ginger)

Day 2:

Breakfast:
- Overnight Chia Seed Pudding with
Mango and Pistachios
- Turmeric Latte (Golden Milk)

Lunch:
- Lentil and Vegetable Soup
- Whole Grain Crackers

- Lemon Water with Fresh Basil

Snack:
- Fresh Fruit Salad with a Drizzle of
Honey

Dinner:
- Grilled Shrimp and Vegetable Skewers
- Brown Rice
- Steamed Asparagus
- Herbal Infusion (Lemon Balm or Mint)

Day 3:

Breakfast:
- Spinach and Feta Omelette
- Whole Grain English Muffin
- Green Tea with Mint

Lunch:
- Chickpea and Spinach Salad with Lemon
Tahini Dressing

- Quinoa Tabouli
- Coconut Water

Snack:
- Hummus with Veggie Sticks (Carrots,
Cucumber, Bell Peppers)

Dinner:
- Teriyaki Tofu Stir-Fry with Brown Rice
- Sautéed Bok Choy
- Herbal Tea Blend (Chai or Lemongrass)

Day 4:

Breakfast:
- Whole Grain Pancakes with Mixed
Berries and Greek Yogurt
- Matcha Green Tea Latte

Lunch:
- Mediterranean Grilled Chicken Wrap
- Tzatziki Sauce

- Infused Water with Citrus Slices

Snack:
- Cottage Cheese with Pineapple Chunks

Dinner:
- Baked Cod with Quinoa and Vegetable
Medley
- Roasted Brussels Sprouts
- Detoxifying Green Tea

Day 5:

Breakfast:
- Berry and Spinach Smoothie Bowl
- Turmeric Ginger Tea

Lunch:
- Quinoa and Black Bean Stuffed Bell
Peppers
- Mixed Greens Salad
- Lemon Water with Fresh Mint

Snack:
- Apple Slices with Almond Butter

Dinner:
- Vegetable Stir-Fry with Tofu and Brown
Rice Noodles
- Ginger Sesame Sauce
- Herbal Infusion (Chamomile or
Peppermint)

Day 6:

Breakfast:
- Oatmeal with Sliced Banana and
Walnuts
- Green Smoothie (Kale, Pineapple,
Coconut Water)

Lunch:
- Tomato Basil Chickpea Pasta
- Mixed Greens Salad

- Lemon Water with Rosemary

Snack:
- Trail Mix (Nuts, Seeds, Dried Fruits)

Dinner:
- Grilled Turkey Breast with Quinoa Pilaf
- Steamed Broccoli
- Herbal Infusion (Lavender or Echinacea)

Day 7:

Breakfast:
- Greek Yogurt Parfait with Mixed Berries and Granola
- Matcha Green Tea

Lunch:
- Lentil and Vegetable Wrap with Whole Grain Tortilla
- Sliced Watermelon
- Infused Water with Basil and Lime

Snack:
- Almond Butter Banana Bites

Dinner:
- Vegetable Curry with Chickpeas and
Basmati Rice
- Sautéed Spinach
- Herbal Infusion (Chamomile or
Lemongrass)

Remember to stay hydrated with water
throughout the day and adjust portions
based on individual needs and
preferences.

Tips for Adapting Recipes to Individual Dietary Needs

The ability to modify recipes to suit unique dietary requirements enables people to enjoy delectable and fulfilling meals while taking into account particular health concerns or personal preferences. The following are some helpful pointers for successfully modifying recipes:

1. Comprehend Dietary Requirements: - Clearly state what kind of diet is required, including for those with allergies, intolerances, certain medical conditions, or personal lifestyle preferences (vegan, vegetarian, or gluten-free).

2. Substitute Ingredients Wisely: - Become familiar with appropriate replacements for ingredients. For example, in gluten-free recipes, use almond or coconut flour instead of wheat flour, or replace dairy milk with soy or almond milk.

3. Try Different Flavours: - Try experimenting with different herbs, spices, and seasonings to bring out the flavours in your food. A dish can be enhanced with fresh herbs and spices without using a lot of sugar or salt.

4. Equilibrium Macronutrients:- Make sure the macronutrient balance in your modified recipes is maintained (carbohydrates, proteins, and fats). For some dietary objectives, this balance can be vital to achieving overall nutrition goals.

5. Portion Control: - Modify serving sizes to satisfy each person's energy needs.

Those who are controlling their blood sugar, weight, or other health issues should pay special attention to this.

6. Mindful Cooking Techniques: - Select cooking techniques that complement nutritional objectives. Instead of frying, try baking, grilling, steaming, or sautéing. These techniques might be appropriate for particular dietary preferences and retain more nutrients.

7. Incorporate Plant-Based Proteins:- Investigate different plant-based protein sources if you're trying to cut back on meat consumption or are on a plant-based diet.

8. Carefully read the labels: Make sure the pre-packaged ingredients you choose meet your dietary requirements by carefully reading their labels. Keep an eye out for substances that are buried and may not be visible right away.

9. Customise Sweeteners:- Try substituting honey, maple syrup, or agave nectar for refined sugars in your recipes. It's especially helpful for people who control their blood sugar levels.

10. Cooking Without Allergens: - Be careful to stay away from allergens if you have allergies. Instead of utilising standard nut butters, think about substituting them with allergy-friendly options like nut or seed butter.

11. Use Whole Foods: - When making modifications, place a strong emphasis on whole, minimally processed foods. These foods help create a balanced and nutritious dict since they frequently hold onto more nutrients.

12. Get Creative with Texture:-
Try experimenting with varied textures by using a range of grains, veggies, and legumes. This can spice up your meals and provide them a more varied range of nutrients.

13. Maintain a Food record:- Keep a food record to monitor your body's reaction to different dietary adjustments. This can assist in spotting trends and directing more modifications.

14. Consult with Professionals: - When in question or handling complicated dietary requirements, speak with certified dietitians or other medical professionals. Personalised advice based on specific medical issues can be given by them.

15. Enjoy the Process: - Accept the adventure of modifying recipes as a fun and imaginative endeavour. It's a chance to sample new flavours and experience the satisfaction of feeding your body in accordance with its own requirements.

Adapting recipes can be a satisfying endeavour that improves one's general well-being and culinary experience when done with consideration and knowledge. These suggestions enable people to enjoy meals that meet their specific dietary requirements, regardless of whether they are motivated by health concerns or personal preferences.

Conclusion

As we approach the conclusion of "Cancer-Fighting Feasts: How to Fight Cancer with Easy and Nourishing Recipes," I would like to express my sincere gratitude to all of our readers for joining us on this gastronomic journey towards health. Your willingness to delve into the world of healthy cuisine shows that you and others are committed to resilience and good health.

We haven't merely focused on recipes in this book; we also want to provide you the tools you need to make thoughtful, health-promoting food decisions. Everything from the kitchen necessities for dishes that fight cancer to delicious breakfasts, healthy lunches, nutrient-dense dinners, and decadent desserts—all created with the intention of feeding your body and soul.

We explored the delectable world of food and nutrition's role in the fight against cancer, giving you a deeper understanding of the significant benefits of mindful eating. We looked at both the "what" and the "why," realising that a comprehensive approach to health requires a grasp of the connection between health and nutrition.

The journey proceeded with helpful advice on customising recipes to meet specific dietary requirements, acknowledging that every person's route to wellness is different. Our goal was to enable everyone, with or without dietary restrictions or preferences, to have access to nutritious, cancer-fighting meals by promoting a flexible and creative approach to cooking.

I invite you to apply the knowledge you have gained from these pages in your own unique way. Try new things in the kitchen, adjust recipes to your preferences, and enjoy the satisfaction of cooking meals that improve your health. Always keep in mind that the journey towards a healthier and more fulfilling life is what matters most, not just the final destination. Enjoy every step of the way.

We appreciate you selecting "Cancer-Fighting Feasts" and putting your faith and time into the idea that delicious food is a potent weapon against cancer in addition to being a source of nourishment. I hope these dishes brighten your table and help you live a long, healthy life full of delightful moments.

With gratitude,

Ryan Stone
Author of "Cancer-Fighting Feasts: How to
Fight Cancer with Easy and Nourishing
Recipes"